This Book is designed to record personal health & physical aspects occurring during your lifetime. Entries should *briefly* record details including Dates, names of practitioners/specialists. Names of Illnesses and information that may be required later in life.

Accuracy of the information, especially dates, is essential to ensure that the data is relevant when filling out important documents such as Insurance applications and other papers which may be medically or Legally contested. (ie Health Insurance)

Ask your medical Practitioner to sign your entries where appropriate.

# MY LIFE
## HEALTH JOURNAL

# MY LIFE
## HEALTH JOURNAL

---

This Book is designed to record personal health & physical aspects occurring
### During your lifetime

## Bob McGarry

**To order additional copies of this book, contact:**
Xlibris Corporation
0800-891-366
www.Xlibris.co.nz
Orders@Xlibris.co.nz
700228

# CONTENTS

## DRUG ALLERGIES

_____

_____

_____

_____

_____

_____

_____

_____

_____

_____

_____

_____

# PERSONAL HEALTH JOURNAL

| **Blood Type** | **Health Board** | **Reference Number** |
| --- | --- | --- |

First Names

Surname 1

Surname 2

Surname 3

Date of Birth                              Time of Birth

**Health Insurer**                        **Policy number**


Address 1


          2



          3



          4



          5



          6



          7

Date              **PERSONAL HEALTH JOURNAL**

## MEDICAL PRACTICES

Contact info

Doctor

Contact info

---

Date

Medical Practice

Contact info

Doctor

Contact info

---

Date

Medical Practice

Contact info

Doctor

Contact info

---

Date

Medical Practice

Contact info

Doctor

Contact info

---

Date

Medical Practice

Contact info

Doctor

Contact info

---

Date

Medical Practice

Contact info

Doctor

Contact info ·

---

# PERSONAL HEALTH JOURNAL

**Next of Kin List**   Include contact phone numbers and address for home & work.

# FAMILY DATA

nclude medical cause of Death
_____

Fathers name
_____

Family medical traits
_____
_____
_____

Mothers Name
_____

Family medical traits
_____
_____
_____

Sisters
_____
_____

Brothers
_____
_____

Schools
_____
_____

Interesting Family Data
_____
_____
_____
_____
_____
_____
_____
_____
_____
_____
_____

## IMMUNISATIONS & ALLERGIES

Date

# PERSONAL HEALTH JOURNAL

RE-OCCURING PROBLEMS

Date

# PERSONAL HEALTH JOURNAL

## JOURNAL ENTRIES INDEX (One-Two words max)

| Page | Page |
|------|------|
| Page | Page |
| Page | Page |
| Page | Page |
| Page | Page |
| Page | Page |
| Page | Page |
| Page | Page |
| Page | Page |
| Page | Page |
| Page | Page |
| Page | Page |
| Page | Page |
| Page | Page |
| Page | Page |
| Page | Page |
| Page | Page |
| Page | Page |
| Page | Page |
| Page | Page |
| Page | Page |
| Page | Page |
| Page | Page |
| Page | Page |
| Page | Page |
| Page | Page |
| Page | Page |
| Page | Page |
| Page | Page |
| Page | Page |
| Page | Page |
| Page | Page |
| Page | Page |
| Page | Page |
| Page | Page |
| Page | Page |
| Page | Page |

# PERSONAL HEALTH JOURNAL

## JOURNAL ENTRIES  INDEX (One-Two words max)

| Page | Page |
|------|------|
| Page | Page |
| Page | Page |
| Page | Page |
| Page | Page |
| Page | Page |
| Page | Page |
| Page | Page |
| Page | Page |
| Page | Page |
| Page | Page |
| Page | Page |
| Page | Page |
| Page | Page |
| Page | Page |
| Page | Page |
| Page | Page |
| Page | Page |
| Page | Page |
| Page | Page |
| Page | Page |
| Page | Page |
| Page | Page |
| Page | Page |
| Page | Page |
| Page | Page |
| Page | Page |
| Page | Page |
| Page | Page |
| Page | Page |
| Page | Page |
| Page | Page |
| Page | Page |
| Page | Page |
| Page | Page |
| Page | Page |

# PERSONAL HEALTH JOURNAL

**JOURNAL ENTRIES INDEX** (One-Two words max)

| Page | Page |
|------|------|
| Page | Page |
| Page | Page |
| Page | Page |
| Page | Page |
| Page | Page |
| Page | Page |
| Page | Page |
| Page | Page |
| Page | Page |
| Page | Page |
| Page | Page |
| Page | Page |
| Page | Page |
| Page | Page |
| Page | Page |
| Page | Page |
| Page | Page |
| Page | Page |
| Page | Page |
| Page | Page |
| Page | Page |
| Page | Page |
| Page | Page |
| Page | Page |
| Page | Page |
| Page | Page |
| Page | Page |
| Page | Page |
| Page | Page |
| Page | Page |
| Page | Page |
| Page | Page |
| Page | Page |

| Date | Briefly record events of significance on 1 line if possible |
|------|-------------------------------------------------------------|
|      |                                                             |

| Date | Briefly record events of significance on 1 line if possible |

Date      Briefly record events of significance on 1 line if possible

| Date | Briefly record events of significance on 1 line if possible |
|------|-------------------------------------------------------------|

| Date | Briefly record events of significance on 1 line if possible |
| --- | --- |

Date      Briefly record events of significance on 1 line if possible

Date        Briefly record events of significance on 1 line if possible

Date　　　Briefly record events of significance on 1 line if possible

Date    Briefly record events of significance on 1 line if possible

| Date | Briefly record events of significance on 1 line if possible |
| --- | --- |

| Date | Briefly record events of significance on 1 line if possible |
| --- | --- |

21

Date      Briefly record events of significance on 1 line if possible

Date      Briefly record events of significance on 1 line if possible

Date      Briefly record events of significance on 1 line if possible

| Date | Briefly record events of significance on 1 line if possible |
|------|-------------------------------------------------------------|

| Date | Briefly record events of significance on 1 line if possible |
|------|------------------------------------------------------------|

| Date | Briefly record events of significance on 1 line if possible |
|------|-------------------------------------------------------------|

**Date**     Briefly record events of significance on 1 line if possible

| Date | Briefly record events of significance on 1 line if possible |
|------|-------------------------------------------------------------|

| Date | Briefly record events of significance on 1 line if possible |
|------|-------------------------------------------------------------|

Date     Briefly record events of significance on 1 line if possible

**Date**  Briefly record events of significance on 1 line if possible

| Date | Briefly record events of significance on 1 line if possible |
|------|-------------------------------------------------------------|

| Date | Briefly record events of significance on 1 line if possible |
|------|-------------------------------------------------------------|

| Date | Briefly record events of significance on 1 line if possible |
|------|-------------------------------------------------------------|

| Date | Briefly record events of significance on 1 line if possible |
|------|-------------------------------------------------------------|

| Date | Briefly record events of significance on 1 line if possible |
|------|-------------------------------------------------------------|

| Date | Briefly record events of significance on 1 line if possible |
|------|-------------------------------------------------------------|

| Date | Briefly record events of significance on 1 line if possible |
|------|-------------------------------------------------------------|

**Date**      Briefly record events of significance on 1 line if possible

ate        Briefly record events of significance on 1 line if possible

Date        Briefly record events of significance on 1 line if possible

Date        Briefly record events of significance on 1 line if possible

| Date | Briefly record events of significance on 1 line if possible |
|------|-------------------------------------------------------------|
|      |                                                             |

| Date | Briefly record events of significance on 1 line if possible |
| --- | --- |

| Date | Briefly record events of significance on 1 line if possible |
|------|-------------------------------------------------------------|

| Date | Briefly record events of significance on 1 line if possible |
|------|------------------------------------------------------------|
|      |                                                            |
|      |                                                            |
|      |                                                            |
|      |                                                            |
|      |                                                            |
|      |                                                            |
|      |                                                            |
|      |                                                            |
|      |                                                            |
|      |                                                            |
|      |                                                            |
|      |                                                            |
|      |                                                            |
|      |                                                            |
|      |                                                            |
|      |                                                            |
|      |                                                            |
|      |                                                            |
|      |                                                            |
|      |                                                            |
|      |                                                            |
|      |                                                            |
|      |                                                            |
|      |                                                            |
|      |                                                            |
|      |                                                            |

| Date | Briefly record events of significance on 1 line if possible |
|------|-------------------------------------------------------------|
|      |                                                             |

Date        Briefly record events of significance on 1 line if possible

| Date | Briefly record events of significance on 1 line if possible |
|------|-------------------------------------------------------------|
|      |                                                             |

| Date | Briefly record events of significance on 1 line if possible |
|------|-------------------------------------------------------------|

| Date | Briefly record events of significance on 1 line if possible |
|------|-------------------------------------------------------------|

ate    Briefly record events of significance on 1 line if possible

| Date | Briefly record events of significance on 1 line if possible |
|------|--------------------------------------------------------------|
|      |                                                              |

Date       Briefly record events of significance on 1 line if possible

Date        Briefly record events of significance on 1 line if possible

| Date | Briefly record events of significance on 1 line if possible |
|------|-------------------------------------------------------------|

| Date | Briefly record events of significance on 1 line if possible |
|------|-------------------------------------------------------------|

| Date | Briefly record events of significance on 1 line if possible |
|------|-------------------------------------------------------------|

Date    Briefly record events of significance on 1 line if possible

| Date | Briefly record events of significance on 1 line if possible |
|------|-------------------------------------------------------------|
|      |                                                             |
|      |                                                             |
|      |                                                             |
|      |                                                             |
|      |                                                             |
|      |                                                             |
|      |                                                             |
|      |                                                             |
|      |                                                             |
|      |                                                             |
|      |                                                             |
|      |                                                             |
|      |                                                             |
|      |                                                             |
|      |                                                             |
|      |                                                             |
|      |                                                             |
|      |                                                             |
|      |                                                             |
|      |                                                             |
|      |                                                             |
|      |                                                             |
|      |                                                             |
|      |                                                             |
|      |                                                             |
|      |                                                             |
|      |                                                             |
|      |                                                             |

**Date**     Briefly record events of significance on 1 line if possible

Date      Briefly record events of significance on 1 line if possible

| Date | Briefly record events of significance on 1 line if possible |
|------|-------------------------------------------------------------|

| Date | Briefly record events of significance on 1 line if possible |
| --- | --- |

Date      Briefly record events of significance on 1 line if possible

Date      Briefly record events of significance on 1 line if possible

| Date | Briefly record events of significance on 1 line if possible |
|------|-------------------------------------------------------------|

**Date**      Briefly record events of significance on 1 line if possible

| Date | Briefly record events of significance on 1 line if possible |
|------|-------------------------------------------------------------|